ALZHEIMER PATIENT

LIKE ME

By Kay W. Nelson

A mistake, but none the less there I was living in a room in Building 5, the Alzheimer's unit. I had driven from South Carolina to Texas, arriving to find my pre-paid efficiency at the active senior unit to be insufficient for my needs. The promised living quarters included a stocked kitchen with refrigerator and stove, bedroom and handicapped shower in the bathroom. To my horror, my scooter couldn't fit in the bathroom. My traveling companion, Cynthia, knowing my intentions to stay a month visiting my family, demanded an immediate solution to my problem. She buzzed from office to office on the four-acre complex situated along the Trinity River. Before I could catch my breath the movers were towing the furniture from my efficiency to another building, which housed the only room available. Cynthia and I sat in an attractive living area outside my new room in Building 5 as the furniture brought the empty room to life. No kitchen, stove or refrigerator, no television, nor radio, just an attractive, small room, nice furniture and most important at that hour, an adequate bathroom. I bid Cynthia farewell and unpacked. Didn't need a kitchen with its conveniences, I thought. The management promised three free meals a day in the dining room.

I opened my eyes that first morning when two uniform-clad women entered my room. Not being a morning person I glared at them, eyes squinted, mouth opened, mind thinking, "Who just entered my private room?" The two ladies said, "We're here to check on you." Fearing I must have slept until noon to have women checking on me I said, "Will you give me a hand, help me to my scooter." I didn't understand why my grogginess left me weak.

Once on the scooter I asked the time. "Almost six," one lady said. My mind couldn't comprehend the events taking place before the rise of the sun. "Could you give me a hand back in bed," I countered. I was told if I needed help to push the button on the necklace put around my neck. Breakfast is from 8:00 to 9:00, they mentioned while leaving my room. I couldn't go back to sleep. I got up, showered and made it to breakfast on time. That's when I realized the only room available, my room, was in the Alzheimer's building.

An interesting threesome, my breakfast buddies. Donna, to my right, said she was afraid to eat in the dining room because one day three big people ran from the kitchen and knocked her and her wheelchair over and she hit her head on the floor. She said the three kept going, didn't even help her get up. Checking her out, I noticed the left side of her body didn't move. A stroke, I thought, but heck, she could have been paralyzed from the three big people that knocked her over. Directly across from me sat Art. He didn't speak. I made a vow to get him to talk before I left. To my left sat a nicely dressed woman named Norma. The food and service were good. Tomorrow I decided I would make an effort to become friends with my assigned dining mates.

After breakfast I planned to drive to my dad's house. On my way out of Building 5, I was stopped by one of the nurses. "Are you a new resident?" she asked.

I explained that I had rented a room in this building for a month to take care of my parents, who were in their 90's. I told her I drove from South Carolina and arrived last night. She gave me a blank stare and faked a smile, nodded her head and said, "How nice." I knew she didn't believe me. I wondered if she would let me escape out the front door to my van. Another patient distracted her and I put my scooter on rabbit and sped through the front door. I clicked the door function to open my van, lowered the ramp, sped up the ramp, closed and locked the door.

My father greeted me in his usual stylish way. He opened the back garage door – the only entrance I could traverse with my scooter – no steps. He asked if he could help me get in, maybe push me or lift the back of my scooter over the little bump that led into the house. I laughed and told him to get out of the way and watch my scooter go. I put the speed on rabbit and zoomed into his home flying over the little bump as if it weren't there. We hugged and I realized again what a gallant man I shared the entire 60 years of my life with. The past two years had slowly taken my dad's sight, balance, hearing, and ability to eat through his mouth. The only nourishment he received was through a tube in his stomach. His bones appeared to be so fragile they might break if I hugged him too hard, weak indeed from the outside but still a giant of a man in his soul. He would have attempted to lift me and my scooter over a mountain if I asked.

"We have hot coffee if you would like," he stated, searching my eyes with his boyish grin.

I made myself coffee and asked to see Betty, my step-mom. She stayed in bed most days. Stage six of Alzheimer's disease kept her confused, and lack -luster. Her personality was sweet and loving for the most part, however, her needs never stopped. And, there were times when she became impossible and hard to deal with.

I went to Betty's room and saw a wilted woman covered in blankets pretending to sleep. I kissed her cheek. She opened her eyes and smiled. "Who are you," she asked speaking slowly, as if her tongue had taken over her mouth and words slurred.

"I'm, Kay, your daughter."

The care givers hadn't arrived yet. There was a three hour break between shifts. I could tell Betty had messed her diaper. I put my hand on Betty's and asked as non-threateningly as possible if I could help her get dressed. She turned over and pretended to sleep again. I gathered her Depends, baby wipes and clothes and again prompted her to let me help her sit. She wouldn't budge. Dad said it's best to wait for Karla, the care giver. I vowed, before I left, to have Betty trust me again. Months lapsed since I saw her last. She had no idea who I was.

That first day at dad's house turned stressful. Karla had gone home and it was about twenty minutes before the next caregiver arrived. Betty slept on the couch in the living room. Dad and I sat at the breakfast room table talking and laughing. Betty appeared at the threshold of the kitchen and pointed to me shaking her finger. "NO, NO, NO," she stammered. Dad and I stood and went over to sooth her. Her words were hard to understand. Dad stepped towards me as I tried talking to Betty. He put his arm around my back and gave me a side hug. Betty got more agitated.

"What is it, dear?" dad implored.

Dad finally understood what she said as she angrily pointed to me. "Girlfriend"

"No," said Dad. "She's not my girlfriend, she's my daughter, you know she was a baby and then she grew up." Dad's gestures mimicked what he spoke. He pretended to hold a baby in his arms rocking it back and forth. Then as he said, "And she grew up," he pointed to me. Betty seemed to get angrier as dad tried to explain.

I went to dad and said, "I'm going to go in the T.V. room until she calms down, she doesn't understand. " Dad feeling distressed touched my shoulder. Loud bangs came from Betty's direction. We both turned to see Betty pounding her clutched fist against the wall. Dad went to Betty's side and took her hands in his. He expressed how much he loved her and didn't want her to hurt herself. I said, "Dad, maybe it's better if you don't touch me and I'll just stay in the other room until Bennye arrives." Betty never quite calmed down.

When the care giver arrived I went to dad and said, "I'm leaving now, don't hug me and don't walk me to my car. I'm just going to sneak out the back. Love you."

Well, my dad is a stubborn man. I don't think anyone's ever left his home without him walking whoever to their car. I maneuvered my scooter around the house to the driveway and there stood dad, by my car. I shook my head from side to side, smiling I said, "You're going to be in trouble." I backed my car out of the driveway and stopped to watch dad walk back to the front door. He staggered, tripped, wiggled and waddled. "God help them." I prayed. The next day I found out Betty had seen dad walk out the front door and locked it behind him. He was stuck out front until the care giver realized what had happened.

On the way back to building 5, I wondered if living in their own house was safe, even with care givers. My siblings had talked about the advantages of nursing homes. My thoughts turned to my living quarters. For a short while life circumstances threw me into a memory care unit. Maybe this was God's way to help me decide if I should push for safer living conditions for my parents. I decided I would stay at the unit for a month and make an informed decision.

I arrived back at Building 5 at 8:00 p.m. Finding the front door locked, I knocked loudly. Two young attendants ran to check out the noise. Although they let me in they advised me to get the code, the doors in Building 5 are locked at 6:00p.m.

The next morning two attendants woke me, again at 6:00 a.m. I told them it wouldn't be necessary to wake me in the future. They smiled and left.

The woman who shared the other side of one of the walls in my room; a lively, spry, tiny woman, talked at length about her dancing, her hair, and how she would be performing at Christmas. I liked her. There didn't appear to be anything wrong with her memory. And, she had a TV. I heard it playing the night before. We could have had a meaningful friendship during my stay except for the fact that every day my sweet neighbor asked where I lived in the building and again told me about her dancing, her hair and her coming Christmas performance.

Without being awakened by attendants at 6:00 a.m., I manage to arrive on time for breakfast the third day of my stay. Donna smiled at me as I sat and she commented on how nice my clothes looked. She told me how her father used to introduce her as the ugly one of his daughters. I protested and told her how pretty she was. She just smiled and said, "You're just being nice." Over the next four weeks I found out during her lifetime she drank alcohol at times and was married twice which produced two children. She feared for her soul because her sister, the perfect Christian, preached to her about drinking and divorce. I finally protested and said her sister was wrong to pretend she knew what God thought of her soul. I told her she was a good, caring, loving person, beautiful inside and out. She started crying; I asked why she cried. She told me it was because I said something bad about her sister. Boy did I feel like a skunk. I tried to retract and start over. Donna finally stopped crying. She always talked about the pain in her leg. She told me Ray, our other breakfast companion, kicked her under the table on purpose. She told me one time she pooped her pants and the poop had eaten away her skin all the way down to her bone. She stated she didn't want to bother the little nurses who would have to clean her. She talked about going back to her home and getting a scooter like mine.

Donna made me smile most of the time and I laughed often at her crazy stories. She told me I made her happy. I noticed she wore the same clothes over and over, clothes that weren't made for winter. She talked of being cold all the time. I learned from the staff she never had visitors and no real support from the outside.

Ray, our other breakfast companion didn't speak, only grunted when I asked him a question. Finally two weeks into my stay he began talking. At first I swelled with pride thinking I coaxed words from his mouth. He said, "You know Norma here," he pointed to Norma, the fourth person who shared our table. I stopped eating and gave him my full attention. He continued, "She's pregnant." Taken back I stammered, "No she isn't," looking in her direction to see how she responded to the remark. Ray continued, "Yes she is and she's a whore." "Oh my I thought." I've awakened a monster. Maybe he did kick Donna under the table?

Norma, was gracious and pretty, wore beautiful clothes and appeared to be the only one of us who had regular visitors to Building 5. I don't know how happy or satisfied she was because it was so difficult for her to put words together.

Another resident I met in Building 5 was a woman who moved in a day after I arrived. I saw the movers bring in beautiful wood furniture, a TV console, refrigerator, paintings, and she shared the other side of my wall. I would have another neighbor with a T.V. I didn't meet her until I came back from my parent's house late in the evening. Ready for bed and while brushing my teeth I heard a loud, frog-like baritone voice screaming, "Help me, please." I left my room, following the voice. I ended up in the new neighbor's room. From her bed she kept screaming, "Help me, please." I asked if she was in pain. "No," she said, "Who are you?" I told her and she said, "I need a nurse." I punched the button to alert a nurse. Two women came to her room and I left. Come to find out she screamed constantly. Every night I woke to her screams. I slept with a pillow over my head which didn't accomplish the job of muffling her screams.

After a week of daily visits to my parents, I found that Betty seemed to look forward to seeing me. To my relief she never remembered thinking I was dad's girlfriend. She even let me help her change her Depends, ONCE. It is awkward helping an adult stand while sitting in a scooter. Guess I inherited my father's stubborn streak. I convinced Betty to sit on the bed. I then instructed her to stand and hold on to my shoulder while I pulled down her dirty underwear. OK. We accomplished that and she fell back on her bed laughing. I held clean Depends in front of Betty and we both tried to put her feet in the correct opening. Betty's feet would move and miss the opening. I have Multiple Sclerosis and I couldn't stand to physically put the feet where they should be. I found myself instructing Betty how to do most of the work. It became a comedy of errors. I started laughing and to my delight she started laughing too. By some miracle we managed to get the underwear and her slacks put together correctly. I brought her the top I selected for her to wear and she put that on herself.

Betty's care giver, Karla, has a magical way of dealing with Betty. When Betty is in a mood and will not cooperate, Karla only has to appear and her soothing voice calms Betty. Once Betty began to cry, big tears rolled down her cheeks. Karla went to Betty's side to find out the reason for the tears. Betty didn't seem to know how to describe her grief. Her hands were in motion but her lips didn't work. Karla gently took Betty's hand and walked her to the bedroom. She told Betty to lie in bed which she did immediately. Karla snuggled in bed beside her and started gently massaging her head and singing a lullaby. Betty stopped crying and tears came to my eyes.

Back at Building 5, I was scooting down the hallway and was stopped by a man who stood in his doorway with a towel over the area where his zipper should be. He said to me "I have a problem, could you come in my room and help me?" I quickly analyzed the situation and said, "I'm not licensed to help you, let me get a nurse," which I immediately did.

Day after day I noticed a routine of behavior from the residents. After breakfast, lunch and dinner, 90% of the residents would return to their rooms. The halls would be empty and doors to rooms closed. By 6:00 p.m. the building looked like a ghost town. The building housed an area for arts and crafts and provided a teacher to help the residents with projects. Occasionally field trips were arranged for those who wanted to leave the confines of the building. I saw a few who took advantage of these opportunities, but the overwhelming majority chose to stay in their rooms behind closed doors.

Most of the nurses and attendants ignored me. I actually began to identify more with the residents of our unit. A lot of the promises made to me up front, in the beginning, that first day, when they changed my room from efficiency to a room in the memory unit, weren't promises that could be kept. I was told my laundry would be taken care of by the staff, my room would be cleaned every week, and if I wanted to eat lunch or dinner in my room all I had to do was call the number that was printed on the menu handed to me, which contained food that could be ordered any time during the day.

Well, none of those promises came to pass simply because there just wasn't a staff big enough to handle the residents in the building, much less me, who didn't need assistance. When I called the number for room service, no one answered. I left my clothes in a basket to be cleaned only to find out there wasn't anyone to do laundry. As for cleaning my room, HA! After two weeks I asked the lady in the office by the front door who washed sheets and cleaned rooms. She didn't have a clue what I talked about.

So, while in the laundry room cleaning my clothes I met my first friend actually on staff. I asked many probing questions and she answered honestly. I found at night there were only three attendants to care for the multitudes of memory-impaired residents in our unit. Most of the attendants were young and I believe earned minimum wage. In my opinion they weren't professional. My screaming neighbor did get on my nerves, but when I heard one of the night attendants come to her room and yell, "Just shut up!" I knew that attendant wasn't the right person for the job.

I told my new staff-friend of the promise made to me by the marketing person for laundry service. She laughed and said there aren't enough people to clean the memory-impaired patients ' rooms. Often laundry is brought in by one person, put in the washer and then left there when the attendant goes off duty. Residents complain of missing clothes all the time. There just aren't enough people to do what needs to be done. I asked about the residents' hygiene, wondering if they are cleaned after an accident in their pants. My staff-friend answered "sadly many residents don't get immediate service in such cases. Also I've seen some of the attendants change the diapers without cleaning feces from the memory impaired resident, leaving sores that cause much pain."

My kids asked why I stayed at the memory unit and why I didn't raise a stink about returning my pre-paid month's rent. They wanted me to move to a hotel where I would feel more comfortable. I wanted to move to a hotel where the grandkids would feel better about visiting. But I was into my mission I told them. I wanted to learn about the care given to people with Alzheimer's disease in assisted care homes. I told them I wanted to know if or if not an assisted living home might be better for Pops and Mimi Betty.

My parents have great insurance and a live-in nursing home would be completely covered. But, they love their home. Unfortunately the price for care givers to live at a private home can deplete a family's finances to the point they have to live from pay check to pay check, or worse. Luckily my father makes a good paycheck, and, yes, he still works. I don't think people in Building 5 have a choice where to live.

The next morning I arrived for breakfast at the appropriate time with a gift for Donna. You see, every morning for two weeks I heard Donna ask to be served V-8 juice. Every morning the attendant on duty says they don't serve V-8 juice. The day before I stopped at the grocery store and bought Donna a big bottle of V-8 juice. I waited until Donna asked, again, for V-8 juice and I pulled the bottle from my purse and asked the attendant to bring a glass with ice. Donna, thrilled and overwhelmed, asked how much she owed me. I told her nothing, I just wanted her to have V-8 juice in the morning. She smiled so big. She said, "You know what I'm going to do for you?" I answered with a surprised, "What?" She said she was going to send a hot toddy to my room that night. I laughed and told her what a treat it will be.

That next weekend I drove to Austin to visit my kids and grandkids. I was on the soccer field watching my three year old grandson learning to play soccer, a class that's designed for his age students. I got a phone call. I answered the I-Phone and it was the director of Building 5. She said she'd gotten reports that I haven't been coming back to my room every night. I told her that was right and said I was on the soccer field in Austin at that moment and wouldn't be in my room that night either. There was a long pause. She then said I would have to sign a release from responsibility when I got back. I laughed, and wondered how I got into my situation.

While I visited Austin I shared some of the stories about living in Building 5 with my children. Eventually, I was asked if any of the men had come on to me.

"What!" I answered.

My education of sexual desires and the elderly, memory deprived adults, began. I refused to believe what I heard. Oh, yes they insisted. Often in nursing homes for Alzheimer's patients, men and women sneak from room to room and have sex. Well, I finally capitulated and informed them in building 5 it wouldn't be hard to go from room to room. There aren't enough attendants to notice an elephant walk down the hall, much less notice a little illicit sex. When I first moved into my room in the building I wasn't given a key. The building looked safe enough. I figured, why lock my door at night? Thinking no one in the residence would be a thief. I never considered they might want a little nookie. I'm telling you, I locked the door to my bedroom when I got back to the memory unit. I also watched and observed for a new type of behavior.

The end of my month at the Alzheimer's unit drew near. I experienced bittersweet feelings. I truly liked some of the residents. My breakfast buddies, for better or worse, became a part of my life. After our breakfast camaraderie that day I went to a hotel before going to dad's home. I reserved a room for another month. I wanted to be with Dad and Betty for Christmas. I felt cheap, like a traitor to my fellow Building 5 refugees. I could leave, they couldn't. They'll never know how much they taught me. I went to dinner that night with, Jennifer my daughter-in-law, and we decided to pool our money and go to a second hand store to buy clothes for Donna. When I delivered the laundered clothes Donna cried and asked me how much she owed me. I said, "Just deliver a hot toddy to my room tonight."

I felt armed with knowledge for my second month in Texas. More relaxed when socializing with Betty, I enjoyed her perhaps more than other times in life. Sounds crazy, but a wonder of God's grace I guess.

Betty's life dealing with Alzheimer's is hell. She's confused, angry at times, unable to express her feelings so she's lost in a world of chaos. She wets and messes her clothes. Soiled spots on her bed and furniture keep us all doing laundry and scrubbing. Dad is confused and feels guilty he can't help. Lord knows he tries. I can see he's tired and frustrated but true to his character, he never complains.

Dad, in advance, gives the care-givers a holiday for Christmas. Lisa, my sister and I decide to cook Christmas dinner. We want this Christmas to be special. The care-giver talked Betty into helping decorate the Christmas tree. When I arrive at Dad's I'm amazed at how festive the house looks a week before Christmas. Dad calls Lisa and me into a huddle. He hands out money saying to buy Christmas presents. I protest and say, I've already bought gifts. He says buy more and throws out names of people who might need a Christmas present. He must have sensed this would be the last Christmas he and Betty would spend on earth.

As a child I remember the flow of Christmas enlivened my spirit. I think this same experience overtook Betty. Instead of sleeping most of the day in her bed she wandered around her home looking at the lights. It wasn't like her nightly, ghostly wandering. These wanderings put a smile on my face as I saw Betty stop, for it seemed like an eternity, to look at the sparkling lights of the Christmas tree. She would punch a button on a stuffed Christmas bear and we would hear a Christmas song. Betty smiled and danced trying to mimic the bear's motions. She would touch us with a beckoning gesture of her hand wanting us to follow where she would continually show us the ever-growing amount of colorful gift wrapped boxes under the Christmas tree. She ate three meals a day. She smiled and laughed at our conversations, though I can't imagine she had a clue what we said.

Christmas day arrived. When I got to the house, breakfast awaited. After breakfast we went to the living room to start the process of opening gifts. Lisa, John and I handed Betty and Dad gift after gift. At first we had to help Betty unwrap the boxes. She laughed when she saw the stuffed animals. Hugging her new cuddly toys, she had to be coaxed to put the gift down and open another box. I loved the motions. Thinking back it might have been the turning of time; I the parent, Betty the child. Dad couldn't believe his bounty. He declared, "I don't believe I've opened so many presents in my entire life." We all experienced a day of joy; a true blessing engulfed us all. I give thanks for those memories.

Arriving back in South Carolina I began a study of Alzheimer's disease. Was there a cure in sight? Alzheimer's is devastating to the person with the illness as well as all who know and love the victim of the illness. It's a personal torture, being lost in the unknown.

I, being the positive thinker, early decided Alzheimer's has allowed individuals to be taken out of this world and deposited into a world of limbo, a world in which God could communicate with special individuals, without the trappings of worldly gimmicks. I still hope this to be the case. I can't imagine any other reason for some to suffer as they do.

One of the most factual and concise articles I read was found in the AARP BULLETIN, for January-February, 2015. The featured article was, THE FACES OF ALZHEIMER'S, Cases are Soaring but Funding Lags. In a nutshell, the article talks about the soaring costs of the disease and the ever-increasing number of cases as our population grows older. The cost of Alzheimer's has surpassed the cost of the treatment for cancer patients and victims of heart disease. Alarmingly, the article talks about the lack of federal funding allotted to the research for the treatment of the disease of Alzheimer's. Washington has committed $5.4 billion to cancer research, $1.2 billion to heart disease, $3.2 billion to HIV/AIDS but only about $566 million in research for Alzheimer's. The article reports Huntington Potter, a neurobiologist at the University of Colorado School of Medicine say, "If we don't get some control over this disease it's going to bankrupt both Medicare and Medicaid."

For my step-mom and my friends in Building 5, there is something that we each can do. We can write our congressional representative. It's only the diseases that have strong political backing that get Federal Funding. Also, for some reason dementia and Alzheimer's are not being talked about loudly enough. The disease is too personal and even the media seems to fail in announcing to the world what's needed for research, and how devastating Alzheimer's can be to a family. Collectively we can stop that by writing our law-makers and politicians. If enough people voice their concerns, the attention will sway Federal Funding. That's what we can do.

The following pages contain the names and phone numbers of members of Congress arranged by state and district in which they serve. A call to your representative will help to draw attention to the number of people who are interested in finding a cure for Alzheimer's. If you are unsure of your district, call the Capitol operator at 202-224-3121. Give the operator the zip code in which you live and the operator will tell you the name of your representative.

Or, while on the phone with your representative's office you can ask for the address of your Congressman or Congresswoman. Then, follow your phone call with a letter.

My father was a member of Congress for 38 years. I know they listen to their constituents. You can make a difference!

Arizona

District	Name	Party	Room	Phone
1	Kirkpatrick, Ann	D	201 CHOB	202-225-3361
2	McSally, Martha	R	1029 LHOB	202-225-2542
3	Grijalva, Raul	D	1511 LHOB	202-225-2435
4	Gosar, Paul A.	R	504 CHOB	202-225-2315
5	Salmon, Matt	R	2349 RHOB	202-225-2635
6	Schweikert, David	R	409 CHOB	202-225-2190
7	Gallego, Ruben	D	1218 LHOB	202-225-4065
8	Franks, Trent	R	2435 RHOB	202-225-4576
9	Sinema, Kyrsten	D	1530 LHOB	202-225-9888

Arkansas

District	Name	Party	Room	Phone
1	Crawford, Rick	R	1711 LHOB	202-225-4076
2	Hill, French	R	1229 LHOB	202-225-2506
3	Womack, Steve	R	1119 LHOB	202-225-4301
4	Westerman, Bruce	R	130 CHOB	202-225-3772

California

District	Name	Party	Room	Phone
1	LaMalfa, Doug	R	322 CHOB	202-225-3076
2	Huffman, Jared	D	1630 LHOB	202-225-5161
3	Garamendi, John	D	2438 RHOB	202-225-1880
4	McClintock, Tom	R	2331 RHOB	202-225-2511
5	Thompson, Mike	D	231 CHOB	202-225-3311
6	Matsui, Doris O.	D	2311 RHOB	202-225-7163
7	Bera, Ami	D	1535 LHOB	202-225-5716
8	Cook, Paul	R	1222 LHOB	202-225-5861
9	McNerney, Jerry	D	2265 RHOB	202-225-1947
10	Denham, Jeff	R	1730 LHOB	202-225-4540

District	Name	Party	Room	Phone
11	DeSaulnier, Mark	D	327 CHOB	202-225-2095
12	Pelosi, Nancy	D	233 CHOB	202-225-4965
13	Lee, Barbara	D	2267 RHOB	202-225-2661
14	Speier, Jackie	D	2465 RHOB	202-225-3531
15	Swalwell, Eric	D	129 CHOB	202-225-5065
16	Costa, Jim	D	1314 LHOB	202-225-3341
17	Honda, Mike	D	1713 LHOB	202-225-2631
18	Eshoo, Anna G.	D	241 CHOB	202-225-8104
19	Lofgren, Zoe	D	1401 LHOB	202-225-3072
20	Farr, Sam	D	1126 LHOB	202-225-2861
21	Valadao, David	R	1004 LHOB	202-225-4695
22	Nunes, Devin	R	1013 LHOB	202-225-2523
23	McCarthy, Kevin	R	2421 RHOB	202-225-2915
24	Capps, Lois	D	2231 RHOB	202-225-3601
25	Knight, Steve	R	1023 LHOB	202-225-1956
26	Brownley, Julia	D	1019 LHOB	202-225-5811
27	Chu, Judy	D	2423 RHOB	202-225-5464
28	Schiff, Adam	D	2411 RHOB	202-225-4176
29	Cárdenas, Tony	D	1510 LHOB	202-225-6131
30	Sherman, Brad	D	2242 RHOB	202-225-5911
31	Aguilar, Pete	D	1223 LHOB	202-225-3201
32	Napolitano, Grace	D	1610 LHOB	202-225-5256
33	Lieu, Ted	D	415 CHOB	202-225-3976
34	Becerra, Xavier	D	1226 LHOB	202-225-6235
35	Torres, Norma	D	516 CHOB	202-225-6161
36	Ruiz, Raul	D	1319 LHOB	202-225-5330
37	Bass, Karen	D	408 CHOB	202-225-7084
38	Sánchez, Linda	D	2329 RHOB	202-225-6676
39	Royce, Ed	R	2310 RHOB	202-225-4111
40	Roybal-Allard, Lucille	D	2330 RHOB	202-225-1766
41	Takano, Mark	D	1507 LHOB	202-225-2305
42	Calvert, Ken	R	2205 RHOB	202-225-1986
43	Waters, Maxine	D	2221 RHOB	202-225-2201
44	Hahn, Janice	D	404 CHOB	202-225-8220
45	Walters, Mimi	R	236 CHOB	202-225-5611
46	Sanchez, Loretta	D	1211 LHOB	202-225-2965
47	Lowenthal, Alan	D	108 CHOB	202-225-7924

District	Name	Party	Room	Phone
48	Rohrabacher, Dana	R	2300 RHOB	202-225-2415
49	Issa, Darrell	R	2269 RHOB	202-225-3906
50	Hunter, Duncan D.	R	2429 RHOB	202-225-5672
51	Vargas, Juan	D	1605 LHOB	202-225-8045
52	Peters, Scott	D	1122 LHOB	202-225-0508
53	Davis, Susan	D	1214 LHOB	202-225-2040

Colorado

District	Name	Party	Room	Phone
1	DeGette, Diana	D	2368 RHOB	202-225-4431
2	Polis, Jared	D	1433 LHOB	202-225-2161
3	Tipton, Scott	R	218 CHOB	202-225-4761
4	Buck, Ken	R	416 CHOB	202-225-4676
5	Lamborn, Doug	R	2402 RHOB	202-225-4422
6	Coffman, Mike	R	2443 RHOB	202-225-7882
7	Perlmutter, Ed	D	1410 LHOB	202-225-2645

Connecticut

District	Name	Party	Room	Phone
1	Larson, John B.	D	1501 LHOB	202-225-2265
2	Courtney, Joe	D	2348 RHOB	202-225-2076
3	DeLauro, Rosa L.	D	2413 RHOB	202-225-3661
4	Himes, Jim	D	1227 LHOB	202-225-5541
5	Esty, Elizabeth	D	405 CHOB	202-225-4476

Delaware

District	Name	Party	Room	Phone
At Large	Carney, John	D	1406 LHOB	202-225-4165

District of Columbia

District	Name	Party	Room	Phone
At Large	Norton, Eleanor Holmes	D	2136 RHOB	202-225-8050

Florida

District	Name	Party	Room	Phone
1	Miller, Jeff	R	336 CHOB	202-225-4136
2	Graham, Gwen	D	1213 LHOB	202-225-5235
3	Yoho, Ted	R	511 CHOB	202-225-5744
4	Crenshaw, Ander	R	2161 RHOB	202-225-2501
5	Brown, Corrine	D	2111 RHOB	202-225-0123
6	DeSantis, Ron	R	308 CHOB	202-225-2706
7	Mica, John	R	2187 RHOB	202-225-4035
8	Posey, Bill	R	120 CHOB	202-225-3671
9	Grayson, Alan	D	303 CHOB	202-225-9889
10	Webster, Daniel	R	1039 LHOB	202-225-2176
11	Nugent, Richard	R	1727 LHOB	202-225-1002
12	Bilirakis, Gus M.	R	2112 RHOB	202-225-5755
13	Jolly, David	R	1728 LHOB	202-225-5961
14	Castor, Kathy	D	205 CHOB	202-225-3376
15	Ross, Dennis	R	229 CHOB	202-225-1252
16	Buchanan, Vern	R	2104 RHOB	202-225-5015
17	Rooney, Tom	R	2160 RHOB	202-225-5792
18	Murphy, Patrick	D	211 CHOB	202-225-3026
19	Clawson,Curt	R	228 CHOB	202-225-2536
20	Hastings, Alcee L.	D	2353 RHOB	202-225-1313
21	Deutch, Ted	D	2447 RHOB	202-225-3001
22	Frankel, Lois	D	1037 LHOB	202-225-9890
23	Wasserman Schultz, Debbie	D	1114 LHOB	202-225-7931
24	Wilson, Frederica	D	208 CHOB	202-225-4506
25	Diaz-Balart, Mario	R	440 CHOB	202-225-4211
26	Curbelo, Carlos	R	1429 LHOB	202-225-2778
27	Ros-Lehtinen, Ileana	R	2206 RHOB	202-225-3931

Georgia

District	Name	Party	Room	Phone
1	Carter, Buddy	R	432 CHOB	202-225-5831
2	Bishop Jr., Sanford D.	D	2407 RHOB	202-225-3631
3	Westmoreland, Lynn A.	R	2202 RHOB	202-225-5901
4	Johnson, Henry C. "Hank" Jr.	D	2240 RHOB	202-225-1605

District	Name	Party	Room	Phone
5	Lewis, John	D	343 CHOB	202-225-3801
6	Price, Tom	R	100 CHOB	202-225-4501
7	Woodall, Robert	R	1724 LHOB	202-225-4272
8	Scott, Austin	R	2417 RHOB	202-225-6531
9	Collins, Doug	R	1504 LHOB	202-225-9893
10	Hice, Jody	R	1516 LHOB	202-225-4101
11	Loudermilk, Barry	R	238 CHOB	202-225-2931
12	Allen, Rick	R	513 CHOB	202-225-2823
13	Scott, David	D	225 CHOB	202-225-2939
14	Graves, Tom	R	2442 RHOB	202-225-5211

Guam

District	Name	Party	Room	Phone
At Large	Bordallo, Madeleine	D	2441 RHOB	202-225-1188

Hawaii

District	Name	Party	Room	Phone
1	Takai, Mark	D	422 CHOB	202-225-2726
2	Gabbard, Tulsi	D	1609 LHOB	202-225-4906

Idaho

District	Name	Party	Room	Phone
1	Labrador, Raul R.	R	1523 LHOB	202-225-6611
2	Simpson, Mike	R	2312 RHOB	202-225-5531

Illinois

District	Name	Party	Room	Phone
1	Rush, Bobby L.	D	2188 RHOB	202-225-4372
2	Kelly, Robin	D	1239 LHOB	202-225-0773
3	Lipinski, Daniel	D	2346 RHOB	202-225-5701
4	Gutierrez, Luis	D	2408 RHOB	202-225-8203

District	Name	Party	Room	Phone
5	Quigley, Mike	D	2458 RHOB	202-225-4061
6	Roskam, Peter J.	R	2246 RHOB	202-225-4561
7	Davis, Danny K.	D	2159 RHOB	202-225-5006
8	Duckworth, Tammy	D	104 CHOB	202-225-3711
9	Schakowsky, Jan	D	2367 RHOB	202-225-2111
10	Dold, Bob	R	221 CHOB	202-225-4835
11	Foster, Bill	D	1224 LHOB	202-225-3515
12	Bost, Mike	R	1440 LHOB	202-225-5661
13	Davis, Rodney	R	1740 LHOB	202-225-2371
14	Hultgren, Randy	R	2455 RHOB	202-225-2976
15	Shimkus, John	R	2217 RHOB	202-225-5271
16	Kinzinger, Adam	R	1221 LHOB	202-225-3635
17	Bustos, Cheri	D	1009 LHOB	202-225-5905
18	LaHood,Darin -- **Vacancy**	R	2464 RHOB	202-225-6201

Indiana

District	Name	Party	Room	Phone
1	Visclosky, Peter	D	2328 RHOB	202-225-2461
2	Walorski, Jackie	R	419 CHOB	202-225-3915
3	Stutzman, Marlin	R	2418 RHOB	202-225-4436
4	Rokita, Todd	R	1717 LHOB	202-225-5037
5	Brooks, Susan W.	R	1505 LHOB	202-225-2276
6	Messer, Luke	R	508 CHOB	202-225-3021
7	Carson, André	D	2453 RHOB	202-225-4011
8	Bucshon, Larry	R	1005 LHOB	202-225-4636
9	Young, Todd	R	1007 LHOB	202-225-5315

Iowa

District	Name	Party	Room	Phone
1	Blum, Rod	R	213 CHOB	202-225-2911
2	Loebsack, David	D	1527 LHOB	202-225-6576
3	Young, David	R	515 CHOB	202-225-5476
4	King, Steve	R	2210 RHOB	202-225-4426

Kansas

District	Name	Party	Room	Phone
1	Huelskamp, Tim	R	1110 LHOB	202-225-2715
2	Jenkins, Lynn	R	1526 LHOB	202-225-6601
3	Yoder, Kevin	R	215 CHOB	202-225-2865
4	Pompeo, Mike	R	436 CHOB	202-225-6216

Kentucky

District	Name	Party	Room	Phone
1	Whitfield, Ed	R	2184 RHOB	202-225-3115
2	Guthrie, S. Brett	R	2434 RHOB	202-225-3501
3	Yarmuth, John A.	D	403 CHOB	202-225-5401
4	Massie, Thomas	R	314 CHOB	202-225-3465
5	Rogers, Harold	R	2406 RHOB	202-225-4601
6	Barr, Andy	R	1432 LHOB	202-225-4706

Louisiana

District	Name	Party	Room	Phone
1	Scalise, Steve	R	2338 RHOB	202-225-3015
2	Richmond, Cedric	D	240 CHOB	202-225-6636
3	Boustany Jr., Charles W.	R	1431 LHOB	202-225-2031
4	Fleming, John	R	2182 RHOB	202-225-2777
5	Abraham, Ralph	R	417 CHOB	202-225-8490
6	Graves, Garret	R	204 CHOB	202-225-3901

Maine

District	Name	Party	Room	Phone
1	Pingree, Chellie	D	2162 RHOB	202-225-6116
2	Poliquin, Bruce	R	426 CHOB	202-225-6306

Maryland

District	Name	Party	Room	Phone
1	Harris, Andy	R	1533 LHOB	202-225-5311

District	Name	Party	Room	Phone
2	Ruppersberger, C. A. Dutch	D	2416 RHOB	202-225-3061
3	Sarbanes, John P.	D	2444 RHOB	202-225-4016
4	Edwards, Donna F.	D	2445 RHOB	202-225-8699
5	Hoyer, Steny H.	D	1705 LHOB	202-225-4131
6	Delaney, John	D	1632 LHOB	202-225-2721
7	Cummings, Elijah	D	2230 RHOB	202-225-4741
8	Van Hollen, Chris	D	1707 LHOB	202-225-5341

Massachusetts

District	Name	Party	Room	Phone
1	Neal, Richard E.	D	341 CHOB	202-225-5601
2	McGovern, James	D	438 CHOB	202-225-6101
3	Tsongas, Niki	D	1714 LHOB	202-225-3411
4	Kennedy III, Joseph P.	D	306 CHOB	202-225-5931
5	Clark, Katherine	D	1721 LHOB	202-225-2836
6	Moulton, Seth	D	1408 LHOB	202-225-8020
7	Capuano, Michael E.	D	1414 LHOB	202-225-5111
8	Lynch, Stephen F.	D	2369 RHOB	202-225-8273
9	Keating, William	D	315 CHOB	202-225-3111

Michigan

District	Name	Party	Room	Phone
1	Benishek, Dan	R	514 CHOB	202-225-4735
2	Huizenga, Bill	R	1217 LHOB	202-225-4401
3	Amash, Justin	R	114 CHOB	202-225-3831
4	Moolenaar, John	R	117 CHOB	202-225-3561
5	Kildee, Daniel	D	227 CHOB	202-225-3611
6	Upton, Fred	R	2183 RHOB	202-225-3761
7	Walberg, Tim	R	2436 RHOB	202-225-6276
8	Bishop, Mike	R	428 CHOB	202-225-4872
9	Levin, Sander	D	1236 LHOB	202-225-4961

District	Name	Party	Room	Phone
10	Miller, Candice	R	320 CHOB	202-225-2106
11	Trott, Dave	R	1722 LHOB	202-225-8171
12	Dingell, Debbie	D	116 CHOB	202-225-4071
13	Conyers Jr., John	D	2426 RHOB	202-225-5126
14	Lawrence, Brenda	D	1237 LHOB	202-225-5802

Minnesota

District	Name	Party	Room	Phone
1	Walz, Timothy J.	D	1034 LHOB	202-225-2472
2	Kline, John	R	2439 RHOB	202-225-2271
3	Paulsen, Erik	R	127 CHOB	202-225-2871
4	McCollum, Betty	D	2256 RHOB	202-225-6631
5	Ellison, Keith	D	2263 RHOB	202-225-4755
6	Emmer, Tom	R	503 CHOB	202-225-2331
7	Peterson, Collin C.	D	2204 RHOB	202-225-2165
8	Nolan, Rick	D	2366 RHOB	202-225-6211

Mississippi

District	Name	Party	Room	Phone
1	Kelly, Trent	R	1427 LHOB	202-225-4306
2	Thompson, Bennie G.	D	2466 RHOB	202-225-5876
3	Harper, Gregg	R	307 CHOB	202-225-5031
4	Palazzo, Steven	R	331 CHOB	202-225-5772

Missouri

District	Name	Party	Room	Phone
1	Clay Jr., William "Lacy"	D	2428 RHOB	202-225-2406
2	Wagner, Ann	R	435 CHOB	202-225-1621
3	Luetkemeyer, Blaine	R	2440 RHOB	202-225-2956
4	Hartzler, Vicky	R	2235 RHOB	202-225-2876
5	Cleaver, Emanuel	D	2335 RHOB	202-225-4535
6	Graves, Sam	R	1415 LHOB	202-225-7041
7	Long, Billy	R	1541 LHOB	202-225-6536

District	Name	Party	Room	Phone
8	Smith, Jason	R	1118 LHOB	202-225-4404

Montana

District	Name	Party	Room	Phone
At Large	Zinke, Ryan	R	113 CHOB	202-225-3211

Nebraska

District	Name	Party	Room	Phone
1	Fortenberry, Jeff	R	1514 LHOB	202-225-4806
2	Ashford, Brad	D	107 CHOB	202-225-4155
3	Smith, Adrian	R	2241 RHOB	202-225-6435

Nevada

District	Name	Party	Room	Phone
1	Titus, Dina	D	401 CHOB	202-225-5965
2	Amodei, Mark	R	332 CHOB	202-225-6155
3	Heck, Joe	R	132 CHOB	202-225-3252
4	Hardy, Cresent	R	430 CHOB	202-225-9894

New Hampshire

District	Name	Party	Room	Phone
1	Guinta, Frank	R	326 CHOB	202-225-5456
2	Kuster, Ann	D	137 CHOB	202-225-5206

New Jersey

District	Name	Party	Room	Phone
1	Norcross, Donald	D	1531 LHOB	202-225-6501
2	LoBiondo, Frank	R	2427 RHOB	202-225-6572
3	MacArthur, Tom	R	506 CHOB	202-225-4765
4	Smith, Chris	R	2373 RHOB	202-225-3765
5	Garrett, Scott	R	2232 RHOB	202-225-4465

District	Name	Party	Room	Phone
6	Pallone Jr., Frank	D	237 CHOB	202-225-4671
7	Lance, Leonard	R	2352 RHOB	202-225-5361
8	Sires, Albio	D	2342 RHOB	202-225-7919
9	Pascrell Jr., Bill	D	2370 RHOB	202-225-5751
10	Payne Jr., Donald	D	103 CHOB	202-225-3436
11	Frelinghuysen, Rodney	R	2306 RHOB	202-225-5034
12	Watson Coleman, Bonnie	D	126 CHOB	202-225-5801

New Mexico

District	Name	Party	Room	Phone
1	Lujan Grisham, Michelle	D	214 CHOB	202-225-6316
2	Pearce, Steve	R	2432 RHOB	202-225-2365
3	Lujan, Ben R.	D	2446 RHOB	202-225-6190

New York

District	Name	Party	Room	Phone
1	Zeldin, Lee	R	1517 LHOB	202-225-3826
2	King, Pete	R	339 CHOB	202-225-7896
3	Israel, Steve	D	2457 RHOB	202-225-3335
4	Rice, Kathleen	D	1508 LHOB	202-225-5516
5	Meeks, Gregory W.	D	2234 RHOB	202-225-3461
6	Meng, Grace	D	1317 LHOB	202-225-2601
7	Velázquez, Nydia M.	D	2302 RHOB	202-225-2361
9	Clarke, Yvette D.	D	2351 RHOB	202-225-6231
10	Nadler, Jerrold	D	2109 RHOB	202-225-5635
11	Donovan, Daniel	R	1725 LHOB	202-225-3371
12	Maloney, Carolyn	D	2308 RHOB	202-225-7944
13	Rangel, Charles B.	D	2354 RHOB	202-225-4365
14	Crowley, Joseph	D	1436 LHOB	202-225-3965
15	Serrano, José E.	D	2227 RHOB	202-225-4361
16	Engel, Eliot	D	2462 RHOB	202-225-2464
17	Lowey, Nita	D	2365 RHOB	202-225-6506
18	Maloney, Sean Patrick	D	1529 LHOB	202-225-5441
19	Gibson, Chris	R	1708 LHOB	202-225-5614
20	Tonko, Paul D.	D	2463 RHOB	202-225-5076

District	Name	Party	Room	Phone
21	Stefanik, Elise	R	512 CHOB	202-225-4611
22	Hanna, Richard	R	319 CHOB	202-225-3665
23	Reed, Tom	R	2437 RHOB	202-225-3161
24	Katko, John	R	1123 LHOB	202-225-3701
25	Slaughter, Louise	D	2469 RHOB	202-225-3615
26	Higgins, Brian	D	2459 RHOB	202-225-3306
27	Collins, Chris	R	1117 LHOB	202-225-5265

North Carolina

District	Name	Party	Room	Phone
1	Butterfield, G.K.	D	2305 RHOB	202-225-3101
2	Ellmers, Renee	R	1210 LHOB	202-225-4531
3	Jones, Walter B.	R	2333 RHOB	202-225-3415
4	Price, David	D	2108 RHOB	202-225-1784
5	Foxx, Virginia	R	2350 RHOB	202-225-2071
6	Walker, Mark	R	312 CHOB	202-225-3065
7	Rouzer, David	R	424 CHOB	202-225-2731
8	Hudson, Richard	R	429 CHOB	202-225-3715
9	Pittenger, Robert	R	224 CHOB	202-225-1976
10	McHenry, Patrick T.	R	2334 RHOB	202-225-2576
11	Meadows, Mark	R	1024 LHOB	202-225-6401
12	Adams, Alma	D	222 CHOB	202-225-1510
13	Holding, George	R	507 CHOB	202-225-3032

North Dakota

District	Name	Party	Room	Phone
At Large	Cramer, Kevin	R	1032 LHOB	202-225-2611

Northern Mariana Islands

District	Name	Party	Room	Phone
At Large	Sablan, Gregorio	D	423 CHOB	202-225-2646

Ohio

District	Name	Party	Room	Phone
1	Chabot, Steve	R	2371 RHOB	202-225-2216
2	Wenstrup, Brad	R	1318 LHOB	202-225-3164
3	Beatty, Joyce	D	133 CHOB	202-225-4324
4	Jordan, Jim	R	1524 LHOB	202-225-2676
5	Latta, Robert E.	R	2448 RHOB	202-225-6405
6	Johnson, Bill	R	1710 LHOB	202-225-5705
7	Gibbs, Bob	R	329 CHOB	202-225-6265
8	Boehner, John A.	R	1011 LHOB	202-225-6205
9	Kaptur, Marcy	D	2186 RHOB	202-225-4146
10	Turner, Michael	R	2239 RHOB	202-225-6465
11	Fudge, Marcia L.	D	2344 RHOB	202-225-7032
12	Tiberi, Pat	R	1203 LHOB	202-225-5355
13	Ryan, Tim	D	1421 LHOB	202-225-5261
14	Joyce, David	R	1124 LHOB	202-225-5731
15	Stivers, Steve	R	1022 LHOB	202-225-2015
16	Renacci, Jim	R	328 CHOB	202-225-3876

Oklahoma

District	Name	Party	Room	Phone
1	Bridenstine, Jim	R	216 CHOB	202-225-2211
2	Mullin, Markwayne	R	1113 LHOB	202-225-2701
3	Lucas, Frank	R	2405 RHOB	202-225-5565
4	Cole, Tom	R	2467 RHOB	202-225-6165
5	Russell, Steve	R	128 CHOB	202-225-2132

Oregon

District	Name	Party	Room	Phone
1	Bonamici, Suzanne	D	439 CHOB	202-225-0855
2	Walden, Greg	R	2185 RHOB	202-225-6730
3	Blumenauer, Earl	D	1111 LHOB	202-225-4811
4	DeFazio, Peter	D	2134 RHOB	202-225-6416
5	Schrader, Kurt	D	2431 RHOB	202-225-5711

Pennsylvania

District	Name	Party	Room	Phone
1	Brady, Robert	D	102 CHOB	202-225-4731
2	Fattah, Chaka	D	2301 RHOB	202-225-4001
3	Kelly, Mike	R	1519 LHOB	202-225-5406
4	Perry, Scott	R	1207 LHOB	202-225-5836
5	Thompson, Glenn W.	R	124 CHOB	202-225-5121
6	Costello, Ryan	R	427 CHOB	202-225-4315
7	Meehan, Pat	R	434 CHOB	202-225-2011
8	Fitzpatrick, Michael G.	R	2400 RHOB	202-225-4276
9	Shuster, Bill	R	2268 RHOB	202-225-2431
10	Marino, Tom	R	410 CHOB	202-225-3731
11	Barletta, Lou	R	115 CHOB	202-225-6511
12	Rothfus, Keith	R	1205 LHOB	202-225-2065
13	Boyle, Brendan	D	118 CHOB	202-225-6111
14	Doyle, Mike	D	239 CHOB	202-225-2135
15	Dent, Charles W.	R	2211 RHOB	202-225-6411
16	Pitts, Joseph R.	R	420 CHOB	202-225-2411
17	Cartwright, Matthew	D	1419 LHOB	202-225-5546
18	Murphy, Tim	R	2332 RHOB	202-225-2301

Puerto Rico

District	Name	Party	Room	Phone
At Large	Pierluisi, Pedro	D	2410 RHOB	202-225-2615

Rhode Island

District	Name	Party	Room	Phone
1	Cicilline, David	D	2244 RHOB	202-225-4911
2	Langevin, Jim	D	109 CHOB	202-225-2735

South Carolina

District	Name	Party	Room	Phone

District	Name	Party	Room	Phone
1	Sanford, Mark	R	2201 RHOB	202-225-3176
2	Wilson, Joe	R	2229 RHOB	202-225-2452
3	Duncan, Jeff	R	106 CHOB	202-225-5301
4	Gowdy, Trey	R	1404 LHOB	202-225-6030
5	Mulvaney, Mick	R	2419 RHOB	202-225-5501
6	Clyburn, James E.	D	242 CHOB	202-225-3315
7	Rice, Tom	R	223 CHOB	202-225-9895

South Dakota

District	Name	Party	Room	Phone
At Large	Noem, Kristi	R	2422RHOB	202-225-2801

Tennessee

District	Name	Party	Room	Phone
1	Roe, Phil	R	407 CHOB	202-225-6356
2	Duncan Jr., John J.	R	2207 RHOB	202-225-5435
3	Fleischmann, Chuck	R	230 CHOB	202-225-3271
4	DesJarlais, Scott	R	413 CHOB	202-225-6831
5	Cooper, Jim	D	1536 LHOB	202-225-4311
6	Black, Diane	R	1131 LHOB	202-225-4231
7	Blackburn, Marsha	R	2266 RHOB	202-225-2811
8	Fincher, Stephen	R	2452 RHOB	202-225-4714
9	Cohen, Steve	D	2404 RHOB	202-225-3265

Texas

District	Name	Party	Room	Phone
1	Gohmert, Louie	R	2243 RHOB	202-225-3035
2	Poe, Ted	R	2412 RHOB	202-225-6565
3	Johnson, Sam	R	2304 RHOB	202-225-4201
4	Ratcliffe, John	R	325 CHOB	202-225-6673
5	Hensarling, Jeb	R	2228 RHOB	202-225-3484

District	Name	Party	Room	Phone
6	Barton, Joe	R	2107 RHOB	202-225-2002
7	Culberson, John	R	2372 RHOB	202-225-2571
8	Brady, Kevin	R	301 CHOB	202-225-4901
9	Green, Al	D	2347 RHOB	202-225-7508
10	McCaul, Michael T.	R	131 CHOB	202-225-2401
11	Conaway, K. Michael	R	2430 RHOB	202-225-3605
12	Granger, Kay	R	1026 LHOB	202-225-5071
13	Thornberry, Mac	R	2208 RHOB	202-225-3706
14	Weber, Randy	R	510 CHOB	202-225-2831
15	Hinojosa, Rubén	D	2262 RHOB	202-225-2531
16	O'Rourke, Beto	D	1330 LHOB	202-225-4831
17	Flores, Bill	R	1030 LHOB	202-225-6105
18	Jackson Lee, Sheila	D	2252 RHOB	202-225-3816
19	Neugebauer, Randy	R	1424 LHOB	202-225-4005
20	Castro, Joaquin	D	212 CHOB	202-225-3236
21	Smith, Lamar	R	2409 RHOB	202-225-4236
22	Olson, Pete	R	2133 RHOB	202-225-5951
23	Hurd, Will	R	317 CHOB	202-225-4511
24	Marchant, Kenny	R	2313 RHOB	202-225-6605
25	Williams, Roger	R	1323 LHOB	202-225-9896
26	Burgess, Michael	R	2336 RHOB	202-225-7772
27	Farenthold, Blake	R	1027 LHOB	202-225-7742
28	Cuellar, Henry	D	2209 RHOB	202-225-1640
29	Green, Gene	D	2470 RHOB	202-225-1688
30	Johnson, Eddie Bernice	D	2468 RHOB	202-225-8885
31	Carter, John	R	2110 RHOB	202-225-3864
32	Sessions, Pete	R	2233 RHOB	202-225-2231
33	Veasey, Marc	D	414 CHOB	202-225-9897
34	Vela, Filemon	D	437 CHOB	202-225-9901
35	Doggett, Lloyd	D	2307 RHOB	202-225-4865
36	Babin, Brian	R	316 CHOB	202-225-1555

Utah

District	Name	Party	Room	Phone
1	Bishop, Rob	R	123 CHOB	202-225-0453
2	Stewart, Chris	R	323 CHOB	202-225-9730

District	Name	Party	Room	Phone
3	Chaffetz, Jason	R	2236 RHOB	202-225-7751
4	Love, Mia	R	217 CHOB	202-225-3011

Vermont

District	Name	Party	Room	Phone
At Large	Welch, Peter	D	2303 RHOB	202-225-4115

Virgin Islands

At Large	Plaskett, Stacey	D	509 CHOB	202-225-1790

Virginia

District	Name	Party	Room	Phone
1	Wittman, Robert J.	R	2454 RHOB	202-225-4261
2	Rigell, Scott	R	418 CHOB	202-225-4215
3	Scott, Robert C.	D	1201 LHOB	202-225-8351
4	Forbes, J. Randy	R	2135 RHOB	202-225-6365
5	Hurt, Robert	R	125 CHOB	202-225-4711
6	Goodlatte, Bob	R	2309 RHOB	202-225-5431
7	Brat, Dave	R	330 CHOB	202-225-2815
8	Beyer, Don	D	431 CHOB	202-225-4376
9	Griffith, Morgan	R	1108 LHOB	202-225-3861
10	Comstock, Barbara	R	226 CHOB	202-225-5136
11	Connolly, Gerald E. "Gerry"	D	2238 RHOB	202-225-1492

Washington

District	Name	Party	Room	Phone
1	DelBene, Suzan	D	318 CHOB	202-225-6311
2	Larsen, Rick	D	2113 RHOB	202-225-2605
3	Herrera Beutler, Jaime	R	1130 LHOB	202-225-3536

District	Name	Party	Room	Phone
4	Newhouse, Dan	R	1641 LHOB	202-225-5816
5	McMorris Rodgers, Cathy	R	203 CHOB	202-225-2006
6	Kilmer, Derek	D	1520 LHOB	202-225-5916
7	McDermott, Jim	D	1035 LHOB	202-225-3106
8	Reichert, David G.	R	1127 LHOB	202-225-7761
9	Smith, Adam	D	2264 RHOB	202-225-8901
10	Heck, Denny	D	425 CHOB	202-225-9740

West Virginia

District	Name	Party	Room	Phone
1	McKinley, David	R	412 CHOB	202-225-4172
2	Mooney, Alex	R	1232 LHOB	202-225-2711
3	Jenkins, Evan	R	502 CHOB	202-225-3452

Wisconsin

District	Name	Party	Room	Phone
1	Ryan, Paul	R	1233 LHOB	202-225-3031
2	Pocan, Mark	D	313 CHOB	202-225-2906
3	Kind, Ron	D	1502 LHOB	202-225-5506
4	Moore, Gwen	D	2245 RHOB	202-225-4572
5	Sensenbrenner, F. James	R	2449 RHOB	202-225-5101
6	Grothman, Glenn	R	501 CHOB	202-225-2476
7	Duffy, Sean P.	R	1208 LHOB	202-225-3365
8	Ribble, Reid	R	1513 LHOB	202-225-5665

Wyoming

District	Name	Party	Room	Phone
At Large	Lummis, Cynthia M.	R	2433 RHOB	202-225-2311